HOW TO LOSE WEIGHT FAST FOR WOMEN

NO MATTER WHERE YOU ARE IN YOUR
JOURNEY, THERE'S NO BETTER
INSPIRATION THAN OTHER WEIGHT LOSS
SUCCESS STORIES.

Kelly Williams

Please note the information contained within this document is for educational and entertainment purposes only. All effort has been executed to present accurate, up to date, and reliable, complete information. No warranties of any kind are declared or implied. Readers acknowledge that the author is not engaging in the rendering of legal, financial, medical or professional advice. The content within this book has been derived from various sources. Please consult a licensed professional before attempting any techniques outlined in this book. By reading this document, the reader agrees that under no circumstances is the author responsible for any losses, direct or indirect, which are incurred as a result of the use of information contained within this document, including, but not limited to, — errors, omissions, or inaccuracies.

TABLE OF CONTENT

YOU CAN DO IT TOO

People want to lose weight for a whole slew of different reasons. Some want to feel better about the way they look and give their self-esteem a boost, while others aim to stop using food as a coping mechanism for emotional struggles. No matter what reasons you have for wanting to shed some pounds or where you are in your journey, these inspiring weight loss success stories prove that it's never too late to turn things around and get a new lease on life. The following people you'll read more about here have battled—and overcome—difficult challenges, such as depression, anxiety, and feelings of self-worthlessness to achieve their weight loss goals. And you know what that means? You can do it, too!

How To Lose Weight fast For Women

The doctor who lost 125 pounds after beating his food addiction

kevin gendreau lost 125 pounds

Courtesy of Kevin Gendreau

Kevin Gendreau, MD, 31, wrestled with a food addiction for more than a decade, and was 306 pounds at his heaviest.

"I was diagnosed with high blood pressure, hypertension, high cholesterol, fatty liver disease, and sleep apnea, among other things," Gendreau told Best Life in October. "I knew they were all because of my eating habits, but I just couldn't stop."

But when his sister was diagnosed with terminal cancer in 2016, it became a wake-up call for him to make his physical health a priority. "What she was going through wasn't her choice," he said. "What I was doing to myself was."

By cutting out all the junk food and replacing it with a diet rich in fruits, vegetables, nuts, and protein, Gendreau lost 125 pounds in 18 months.

"The best advice that I can give is to find a motivation to change," he said. "For me, it was my sister getting sick and needing to be there for her kids, but it could be anything. Once you find that reason and commit to it, you're good to go."

The 73-year-old woman who lost 55 pounds and became a viral sensation

joan macdonald loses 55 pounds

Joan MacDonald/Instagram

Think it's too late to change your body once you're over 50? Think again. In October, 73-year-old Joan MacDonald became an internet inspiration after showing off her incredible transformation.

"For many decades, I was more often overweight than at a healthy weight," MacDonald told The Daily Mail. "I was on medication for high blood pressure, high cholesterol, and acid reflux. My arthritis was acting up pretty bad."

Concerned about her health, MacDonald's daughter taught her mom how to use her iPhone to track her meals and exercise activity. That tool helped drive her to eat more protein and healthy fats, and go to the gym four or five days a week. And after making those major changes to her lifestyle, MacDonald lost 55 pounds in a year, gained plenty of muscle, and now helps others reach their fitness goals, no matter how old they are.

"For those who truly feel at a loss, I'd say change one thing with your food intake, one exercise to do, and each week add something new," she said. "Don't expect miracles right away, take it slow and steady but keep building."

The woman who lost 190 pounds after overcoming an eating disorder

Amber Neal lost 190 pounds

Amber Neale/Instagram

Amber Neale spent most of her young-adult life in a pattern of losing weight on various diets, and then gaining it all back. In January 2017, she hit 325 pounds—her second heaviest weight—and decided to seek treatment from a mental health professional to address her unhealthy eating habits.

"I realized I needed help when I found myself living the same dismal day over and over again—and food was my only oasis," Neale told Women's Health in April 2019. "It took therapy to make me realize how awful my eating habits had become: I ate from the moment I woke up to the moment I went to bed."

Once she dealt with her anxiety, depression, and binge-eating disorder, Neale was able to cut out fast food, reduce her portion sizes, and start exercising daily for 45 minutes. She lost 190 pounds in two years, and today, she says she takes things "one meal, or one moment, at a time."

The man who lost 150 pounds thanks to his college professor

Joey Morganelli/Instagram

When Joey Morganelli was 16 years old, he watched his father die of a heart attack right in front of him, only three years after losing his mother to cancer. Looking for a way to cope with such tragedy and loss, he turned to food. By the time he graduated high school, he weighed 400 pounds.

Luckily, Morganelli had people around him who cared about his wellbeing and were concerned by what they saw. In his freshman year of college, his microbiology professor pulled him aside to express concerns about his health, and asked him to watch the 2011 documentary Fat, Sick and Nearly Dead. The film had a major effect on Morganelli and slowly but surely, he replaced fast food with healthy, home-cooked meals. Eventually, he became more committed, going on a vegan diet, and by mid-2018, he had lost 150 pounds.

In January 2019, he wrote on Instagram that even though losing weight is hard, what's harder is facing yourself and dealing with the issues that drove you to overeat to begin with. "Give yourself a fair fight and take that blindfold off," he wrote. "It will propel you into places you never thought you could be."

The woman who became a fitness influencer after giving up alcohol

JellyDevote/Instagram

We all know alcohol contains plenty of calories, has little nutritional value, and can impede weight-loss and other lifestyle goals we set for ourselves. But a viral post by Instagram influencer Jelly Devote really showed just how much curbing heavy alcohol consumption in favor of drinking more water can help you lose weight.

The photo on the left shows her at 21, during her college partying days, when she was drinking beer and cider with abandon. Now 27, Devote exercises, drinks in moderation, and feels like she's aging in reverse as a result.

"I'm a new person and I feel better both on the inside and about my outside," she wrote on Instagram in February.

The bride who lost 135 pounds and wore her dream wedding dress

Mary Jane O'Toole/Instagram

When Mary Jane O'Toole got engaged to her longtime boyfriend in 2016, she couldn't have been more excited about it. Weighing 281 pounds, however, made picking out a wedding dress somewhat of a disheartening process.

"I didn't want to buy a plus-size wedding dress, because they cost way more than straight sizes," O'Toole told People in April. "I felt like I was paying this fat tax—I didn't have the ability to buy affordable clothes because I was bigger."

When she and her husband-to-be saw photos of themselves from a trip to Disney World, they made the decision to lose weight together and began tracking their calories and meals with the the app LoseIt!

O'Toole lost 75 pounds in the first year, and another 25 once the couple began incorporating exercise into their routine. By the time the wedding rolled around earlier this year, she had lost a total of 135 pounds and was able to walk down the aisle in the dress of her dreams.

The teen who lost 175 pounds and fell in love with fitness

Hunter Croteau/Instagram

Hunter Croteau had to go to the doctor to find out he was 367 pounds, because the scale at his home was no longer capable of weighing him. Once he graduated high school and with the help of his family, Croteau threw himself into a healthy diet. But two weeks in, he fell off the wagon.

"I knew lying in bed that night that I was not going to go back on the diet the next morning, and I needed to make a drastic step," Croteau told Yahoo! Lifestyle in July. His doctor suggested getting sleeve gastrectomy, which typically removes 80 percent of the stomach and therefore limits the amount of food a person can consume.

Croteau decided to have the surgery, even though he was "extremely nervous" going into the operation. "You're going into this building specifically because you're fat," he said. "It's almost like you're coming to terms with it in front of the world. You're saying, 'I need help. I can't do this on my own.'"

About a month after the surgery, Croteau began going to the gym, and he became increasingly interested in the science of fitness. Thanks to his workout routine and portion control, he lost 175 pounds in eight months and is now studying to become a certified personal trainer.

While he believes that the surgery was "totally worth it," Croteau also credits his love of exercise with helping him keep the weight off and stay in shape. "You need to fall into a habit of something you can maintain, something you enjoy," he said.

The woman who lost 220 pounds for her health

Stacy Blair/Instagram

By the time she was 28, Stacy Blair was already beginning to have health problems due to her weight.

"I was taking medication for high blood pressure, my asthma was getting worse, and it was physically painful to walk or stand for more than five minutes," Blair told Women's Health in October.

For the first time in her life, she was motivated to lose weight not for the sake of looking good, but for personal wellness and improving her health—an approach that changed everything.

"I wanted to be able to play an active role in my little brothers' lives rather than watching from the couch," she said. "I wanted to be able to be a mom one day. I wanted to be able to move without being in pain. I wanted to live instead of just exist."

Blair got started by counting calories and keeping a daily log of her meals, which led to her going on a keto diet that helped her lose 220 pounds in 17 months.

"At the end of the day when everything is all said and done, it's not about the weight you lose, it's about the life you gain," she said.

The mom who lost 80 pounds and discovered self-care

Stacey Welton, 50, knew she'd never be a gym aficionado—not with six kids and a full-time job as a teacher, at least. But once her weight began to give her health problems, she knew something had to give.

"I saw a picture of myself and wasn't happy," Welton told Best Life in July. "I knew that, as I was getting older, that the weight would continue to increase if I did nothing, so I made up my mind to change my life once and for all."

She went on the Atkins diet, which had her eating fewer carbs—and in just eight months, she shed 80 pounds.

"I learned to eat to live, not live to eat," Welton said. "I would say that weight loss is one of the very few areas where it's OK to be selfish. It is about you. Whatever it costs, it's worth the personal investment in you. This is the sacrifice that a mom has to make—not only for herself, but her family."

The man who lost 90 pounds with the help of his girlfriend

Jared Sklar/Instagram

As a kid, Jared Sklar loved to play sports. But when the 27-year-old fell in love with his girlfriend, Samatha MacDonald, he gained some relationship weight. All those late nights spent snacking on the couch with his parter left him at 285 pounds, and when he opened up his refrigerator one day and saw pizza boxes from four different restaurants, he decided something had to change.

"It's pretty embarrassing, but it's the truth," Sklar told CNN in August. "I just opened the door, and I was just like, 'What are we doing here?'"

Sklar and MacDonald decided to give intermittent fasting a try, eating all of their meals between noon and 8 p.m. They immediately noticed that their energy levels increased, and with even more of a drive to be active, the couple used the buddy system to go to the gym six days a week for 45 minutes of indoor cycling.

"We pushed each in our weak areas," MacDonald said. "We were on different pages initially but pushed each other to be on the same page, and that was a huge help."

MacDonald lost 12 pounds, and said that the mental health benefits of going to the gym are the real win for her. Meanwhile, Sklar lost 95 pounds in about seven months, and is now a fitness instructor teaching indoor cycling classes.

"It was hugely beneficial to have a support system with me," he said. "There are always going to be those days where you want to cheat and have a pizza, and just having a support system to keep you in check and being responsible for keeping somebody else in check was really important to me."

The mom who lost 76 pounds and became a wellness coach

JenniferRiviera/Instagram

At nearly 200 pounds, Jennifer Riviera no longer had the energy to play with her 13-year-old son—and her weight was also taking a toll on her marriage.

"My husband and I weren't getting along because frankly, I made it really hard to love me because I stopped loving myself," Riviera told People in August. "Everybody became more important than I did and fast food became my way of life."

Then, two years ago, she saw a friend post about her weight loss journey and found it inspiring. Her friend recommended Isagenix— a dietary supplement brand that makes meal replacement shakes. Now 115 pounds, Riviera is a full-time health and wellness coach who loves yoga. She says she continues to drink at least one Isagenix shake per day and, most importantly, she now has the energy to play with her son.

The man who lost 150 pounds thanks to math deandre weight loss story

Deande Upshaw/Instagram

At 6'7" and 400 pounds, DeAndré Upshaw was a big presence in any room he walked into. And while he loved the spotlight and didn't necessarily hate the way he looked, the 30-year-old knew that his weight could pose certain health risks as time went on. So, rather than going on some of the fad diets that he had experimented with in the past, Upshaw began doing more math and started meticulously counting calories. "The coolest thing about calories in, calories out is that it was math," he told Men's Health in January.

He also avoided escalators and elevators, and used a Fitbit to ensure that he took at least 10,000 steps a day. As a result, Upshaw lost 150 pounds in just one year, and now, he hopes to inspire others to put in the hard but rewarding work it takes to make a weight loss transformation. "I didn't lose 150 pounds once," he said. "I lost one pound 150 times."

The woman who lost 135 pounds on her own terms

Vanessa Flores/Instagram

Growing up, Vanessa Flores was always overweight. She tried several fad diets to slim down, but nothing stuck—a vegan diet helped her lose 60 pounds but proved difficult to maintain. But when she switched to a low-carb diet, which allowed her to have more carbs on days when she worked out, it was a whole different story. Since making that lifestyle change in 2013, Flores has lost 135 pounds, and she's still going.

"I think I started my weight loss journey for the wrong reasons," she told Women's Health in January. "Deep down, I just wanted a boyfriend and wanted to be prettier. But since then, I've realized my weight loss means so much more than that. I've not only gained more confidence, but I feel healthier than ever. Now, I feel like I can do anything—in a relationship or not."

The woman who lost 101 pounds after being turned down from an amusement park ride

Sophie Trewick/Instagram

By the time Sophie Trewick, 23, was in college, she weighed 331 pounds. But a 2017 trip to an amusement park was the last straw for the co-ed. "The staff at the theme park gave us all fast track passes so I didn't have to queue to see if I'd fit on each rollercoaster," Trewick told The Daily Mail in April. "One of my friends actually said to me 'I am glad you are fat as we get to jump straight to the front.' I went home that day distraught, and knew I had to change."

She cut out the junk food, began exercising three times a week, and joined the UK weight-loss organization Slimming World. According to a recent Instagram post, she's lost 101 pounds since 2017.

The woman who lost 150 pounds despite her thyroid condition

Desiree Alexis-Kae Mize/Instagram

When she was eight years old, Desiree Alexis-Kae Mize was diagnosed with hypothyroidism—a condition that affects approximately three million Americans and causes a variety of symptoms, including a slow metabolism. Remaining active often helped her lose weight, but eventually she'd gain it all back. By 21, Mize weighed 260 pounds, and her doctor suggested gastric bypass surgery, which would reduce the size of her stomach, making it easier to practice portion control.

At first, Mize felt like getting surgery would be the easy way out, but she decided to go through with it after hearing the inspiring success stories of women whose lives were changed by the procedure.

"I also learned that the surgery would help me with portion control, but my weight-loss would still require the discipline that I'd been working on my entire life," she told Women's Health in April. "The only difference was this time, I'd actually see results."

A year after the surgery, Mize has lost 150 pounds and continues to exercise and maintain a healthy diet. While the surgery got the ball rolling, it's been her responsibility to keep it moving forward, and she's proud to be doing the work.

"I feel like I'm finally happy and confident with myself and my body," she said. "I know gastric bypass surgery isn't the best choice for everyone, but it was the right choice for me, and it definitely wasn't the 'easy way out.' It not only helped me see results I never thought were possible because of my health condition—but it has also helped me stay healthier by keeping my weight in check."

The man who lost over 100 pounds and became a bodybuilder

Quantel Thomas/Instagram

Many of us wake up on New Year's Day with the resolution to lose weight and get fit. But Quantel Thomas actually did it. Overweight since childhood and 300 pounds by the time he was 18, Thomas kicked off 2017 by starting a routine that found him at the gym six days a week, helping him to lose 180 pounds in 10 months.

Now weighing 204 pounds, he continues his bodybuilding and fitness regimen, and can bench press 285 pounds and deadlift up to 475 pounds. "To be able to love myself, that's the true, ultimate milestone achieved to this day," Thomas told Men's Health in November.

The woman who lost 80 pounds and became a social media influencer

randi vasquez lost 80 pounds

Randi Vasquez/Instagram

Randi Vasquez always struggled with her weight, but it never really bothered her until she got out of her "post-grad slump" in 2014 and realized her boozy brunches and weekend binges had brought her up to 240 pounds.

"I stared at myself in the mirror with tears in my eyes and asked myself, 'How did I let myself get like this?" Vasquez told Women's Health in March. "I always tried to blame it on my genes, but really, I was obsessed with fast food and I wasn't working out."

She kept trying to adopt healthier eating habits, and while she did lose some weight, it wasn't nearly as much as she wanted. Then her friend recommended Kayla Itsines' Bikini Body Guide program. From the first 28-minute workout, she was hooked.

"It was never easy, but I saw my body and mindset change so much and that kept me going," she said. "For the first time ever, I totally believed in myself and knew that I was capable of my weight loss goals." Her fitness regime inspired her to eat healthy, too. She does the Whole 30 diet when she falls off track and needs to get back to good patterns. All in all, Vasquez has lost 80 pounds, and gained more than 70,000 Instagram followers in the process.

"I've gotten out of my comfort zone and experienced a whole life that I never thought

I'd be a part of," she recently wrote on Instagram. "While my belly may be a little fluffier today, I'm happy from where I started and eager to see where I'll end up."

The dad who lost 92 pounds to be a better father

Jeremiah Peterson/Instagram

In 2017, Jeremiah Peterson, 40, went on a hiking trip with his family and quickly found that he couldn't keep up with his young children.

"I had a kind of 'aha' moment," Peterson told The New Haven Register in April. "I reflected on what my life had been. I thought about what my life was at that very moment, and saw what I wanted my life to be."

At the time, his days were consumed by the antiques store he had opened with his wife, and his evenings were spent sitting around drinking beer. Weighing 290 pounds at the time, he decided to make some changes by going on the keto diet, cutting out all alcohol, and hiking in the great outdoors. Once he was in better shape, he began lifting weights again, and his body transformation has garnered him more than 113,000 Instagram followers. He certainly looks like he could run after his kids without losing his breath now.

"The road to your dreams isn't always going to be easy to accomplish," Peterson recently wrote on Instagram. "Just remember this if you get lost along the way: that anything worth having doesn't come easy. You have to be willing to dig down deep and do the work and most importantly never give up."

The A-list celebrity who lost the baby weight

Jessica Simpson/Instagram

Back in May 2017, Jessica Simpson had an awkward interview on Ellen, in which she quashed pregnancy rumors related to her weight gain. The proud mother of three has frequently been the subject of vicious tabloid headlines mocking her post-kids physique. So in September, she rocked the internet when she revealed that she had "tipped the scales at 240" and was "100 pounds down" just six months after giving birth to her third child.

"[I'm] so proud to feel like myself again," Simpson wrote on Instagram. "Even when it felt impossible, I chose to work harder."

Weight Loss? Don't Do This!

Ask anyone who's ever attempted to drop a few pounds and they'll tell you: Losing weight isn't easy. And it certainly doesn't help that the best way to do it isn't so clear-cut. It seems like there's a new diet scheme or exercise trend making headlines every day, promising to help you slim down faster than ever. Sure, some weight loss plans are genuine breakthroughs, but others are full of dubious, if not totally unsubstantiated, advice. So, before you make your plan to lose weight, it's best to get a handle on which recommendations you should outright ignore. To help you weed out what not to do, we talked to nutritionists, fitness experts, dietitians, and other medical experts to pull together the definitive list of unhealthy weight loss tips you should avoid at all costs.

1

Exercise is the be-all and end-all.

"There's too much emphasis placed on workouts as the answer to weight loss," says Ariane Hundt, MS, a New York-based clinical nutrition coach and fitness expert. Although working out will initially promote weight loss, she says, the body "adapts to everything," and the amount of calories burned in a given workout will steadily decline. While Hundt admits that exercise is essential insofar as it helps to maintain muscle mass during weight loss, it can "only do so much" unless it is coupled with a reduced-calorie diet.

2

You need to exercise and diet at the same time to lose weight.

Despite being "recommended by every single diet program out there," Hundt says that "the combo of eating less and exercising more will at some point create intense hunger … and lower your energy." In effect, the combination cancels itself out over time, and it can "only work for so long," she explains.

Instead, try switching up your exercise and diet plans to match your primary focus. For example, "if you want to eat less, you should down-regulate the intensity of your workouts," Hundt says. Conversely, if you want to train for a marathon, "the energy requirements will shift upwards" and you should add more protein and vegetables to your meals.

3

Low-carb diets are a good way to slim down.

Of course, you're familiar with the Atkins diet and the current craze, the keto diet. But while plans like these may move the numbers on the scale immediately, they're generally not helpful for long-term success. "Low-carb diets are not always terrible, especially if they cut out added sugar and processed carbohydrates. However, whole grains, fruits, vegetables, nuts, and beans all have carbohydrates and lots of other nutrients like fiber," explains ACSM-certified exercise physiologist Melissa Morris. "A low-carb diet can cause short-term rapid weight loss, but it's usually water weight. If you plan on eating carbs again, that weight will come back on."

4

And low-fat diets help with weight loss, too.

Low-fat diets are just as bad as low-carb diets when it comes to weight loss. "Fat consumption leads to satiety, which allows you to feel more full for longer and reduces overeating," explains holistic nutrition expert Kyria Marie, MA. "Consequences of a low-fat diet include the following: poor brain function, compromised heart health, low energy, hormonal imbalance, overeating, higher risk of diabetes and depression, and, of course, weight gain."

5

Fat makes you fat.

Don't be afraid of incorporating healthy fats into your diet. Fat in your diet doesn't always mean fat on your body. And according to Marie, good sources of fat like "avocados, olives, coconuts, pastured eggs, nuts, seeds, and small amounts of high-quality meat and seafood" are all "essential for energy, cell growth, and balanced hormones."

6

Significantly reducing calories will increase weight loss.

The danger of reducing caloric intake too quickly is that it sends your body into "starvation mode," explains Morris. "Any diet that cuts calories drastically will actually do more harm than good because your body will start to think it is starving and slow metabolism to compensate for this," she says. "A slower metabolism means fewer calories burned throughout the day, which is not good for weight loss."

With a severe caloric deficit, your body is unsure it will be getting any nutrients in the near future, and so begins to burn muscle— along with fat—to compensate. In addition, the body begins to store future caloric intake as fat so as to prevent it from feeling "starved" ever again.

7

All calories are created equal.

Because calories are described numerically, it can seem as if 100 calories of one snack is equal to 100 calories of another. However, when it comes to weight loss, this simply isn't true.

"While numerical values may be the same, little else is the same when it comes to the calories between an avocado and a cookie. The combination of other nutrients in any food play a role in the reactions it triggers in the body," explains personal trainer and certified nutrition coach Candice Seti, PsyD. "Sugary foods, highly processed foods, and the like—even those low in calories—trigger inflammatory reactions in the body, promote cravings, and deprive the body of much-needed macronutrients."

8

Eating an all-protein diet will help you lose weight fast.

Protein is an important part of every meal plan. However, an all-protein diet is not going to do you any favors. "Your body needs other nutrients and vitamins to survive and thrive," according to weight loss doctor David Nazarian, MD, and nutritionist Desiree Nazarian, MPH, of Weight Loss Clinic Los Angeles. They say that eating an all-protein diet "will lead to a variety of other problems down the line."

9

Prolonged periods of fasting are good for weight loss.

There is a difference between intermittent fasting—which involves eating within a specific time frame—and unintentionally starving yourself by skipping meals. "Our bodies and digestive track are setup to eat multiple times a day. Long periods of fasting can put you in danger and rob you of essential vitamins, minerals, and nutrients that our body needs," the Nazarians explain.

10

You have to work out every day to lose weight.

There's no need to place undue stress on yourself for missing a day at the gym. In fact, incorporating rest days and active recovery days into your schedule is encouraged to promote healing, growth, and recovery.

"Although exercise is important to incorporate into a healthy lifestyle, overexercising can lead to sleeplessness, [as well ass] cardiovascular, musculoskeletal, and mental health issues," the Nazarians explain. "In general, anything extreme in the realm of weight loss is not sustainable and not healthy."

11

Consuming large amounts of caffeine can help you lose weight.

Caffeine does have appetite-suppressing effects. However, the Nazarians explain that "large amounts of caffeine can be dangerous." When consumed in excess, caffeine "can cause decreased absorption and metabolism of calcium, which can lead to osteoporosis."

12

Liquid diets are an effective weight loss tool.

A liquid diet or cleanse is far from necessary if you're looking to lose weight. On the contrary, it's actually pretty bad for you.

"Juice cleanses are often thought of as a way to detox your body and lose a few pounds. However, the negative side of juice cleanses is that it is all carbohydrates, which impacts your blood sugar levels significantly," explains NASM-certified fitness nutrition specialist Renata Trebing of Nourish with Renata. "You have a sudden boost of carbs and an increase in blood sugar, then an energy crash once your insulin kicks in. This leaves you feeling lethargic, moody, and, worst of all, hangry!"

13

Going vegan will increase your weight loss.

Eliminating animal products can make it more difficult to remain satiated and maintain energy levels. So, while "cutting out entire food groups may make you feel good about the label of being 'vegan,'" Hundt notes that finding "what works for you is the best thing you can do to see changes that last a lifetime."

14

You have to eat between meals to keep your metabolism stoked.

While many people believe that you need to eat almost constantly to keep your metabolism running like a well-oiled machine, that's far from the truth. According to a 2017 study published in The Journal of Nutrition, eating less often and spacing out your meals is actually the most effective method for long-term weight loss. To keep your metabolism constantly working, try gaining muscle mass, which Hundt refers to as "your body's furnace."

15

You can't snack and lose weight.

If you are a snacker though, worry not. While snacking all day long isn't going to help you reach your weight loss goals, that doesn't mean you need to abstain completely. In fact, research published in 2012 in the Journal of the American Dietetic Association suggests that snacking may be an easy way to enjoy more healthy foods and stave off hunger. Instead of "to snack or not to snack," the question should really be what to snack on.

16

You have to give up alcohol to lose weight. Cutting back on alcohol—especially if your intake levels are high—can certainly help you lose weight. But the idea that there needs to be a blanket ban on all alcohol is misguided. For example, in a 2013 study published in the Journal of the American College of Nutrition, the addition of two glasses of red wine along with dinner "did not appear to influence" participants' weight gain in either direction. So feel free to drink in moderation.

17

You can't eat after 8 p.m. if you want to slim down.

"There is nothing magical about 8 o'clock," says registered dietitian Adrianne Delgado, nutrition manager at BodyMetrix, LLC. "I'm more concerned with what you eat—and how much—than when you eat."

18

You have to exercise first thing in the morning to lose weight.

Though working out first thing in the morning might give you more energy and start your day off on the right note, Delgado says that "you can be successful working out any time of the day." If your mornings are way too busy to even fathom fitting in a workout, then go ahead and hit the gym at night. At the end of the day, it's the fact that you're moving that matters.

19

You'll lose more weight if you exercise after fasting.

The combination of fasting and exercise is probably not the magic bullet for weight loss you're hoping for. In a 2011 paper published in the Strength and Conditioning Journal, certified strength and conditioning specialist Brad Schoenfeld notes that exercising after fasting induces the breakdown of muscle mass, making it ineffective for those seeking a lean, toned physique.

20

You need to work out longer to see weight loss results.

While many exercisers believe they need to push themselves to the limit at every workout, that's simply not the case. In fact, doing so can be harmful, putting you at increased risk for injury over time. According to a 2018 study published in the Journal of the American Heart Association, it simply doesn't matter how long each individual workout is, as long as the same amount of exercise is accumulated over time.

21

You have to give up natural sugar to slim down.

Avoidance of sugar is a staple of many diets, but these plans go too far when they advise the avoidance of natural sugars, too. In one 2003 study published in the journal Nutrition, participants who consumed three apples— which are full of natural sugar—each day actually lost more weight than those who consumed an oat-based snack.

22

Skim milk is always better than full-fat.

Think sticking to skim milk will help you slim down? Think again. In a 2016 study of more than 18,000 women published in the American Journal of Clinical Nutrition, women who consumed full-fat dairy were 8 percent less likely to be obese than those who opted for skim.

23

Artificial sweeteners are good for weight loss.

While an artificial sweetener will indeed have fewer calories than its sugary counterpart, simply substituting one for the other won't do the trick when it comes to weight loss. Since artificial sweeteners mimic the taste of real sweeteners, they only serve to maintain sugar cravings and dependence, according to a 2010 study in the Yale Journal of Biology and Medicine. So, leave those Splenda packets where you found them.

24

Switching to diet soda is a good weight loss move.

Diet soda might have fewer calories, but because of those artificial sweeteners, it's not really better for your waistline. "Diet soda is filled with artificial sweeteners that are harmful to your body. They also prevent your brain from correctly regulating appetite, causing you to consume more food," explain the Nazarians.

25

Cardio is the only way to burn fat.

Cardio is great for your heart, your mind, and your body, but that doesn't mean it's the only way to slim down. "While cardio is great for your heart health, it isn't the best workout to maximize calories burned," explains nutrition coach and personal trainer Kristin Foust. "Exercise that involves lifting weights is the best workout to add, as muscles continue to burn calories after the workout ends for up to 48 hours. In cardio, that [calorie-burning] period is much shorter."

26

You can target specific areas where you want to trim down during your workouts.

Unfortunately, it isn't possible to target specific areas–like your arms or abs—during a workout. "While you can gain muscle in specific areas, you can't control where your body loses fat. You have to focus on nutrition to see desired fat loss," Foust explains.

27

Certain foods have negative calories.

While there are many foods that are low in calories—celery and lemons, for example—no food has a negative caloric impact. Though it is theoretically possible that the energy needed to digest a food could be greater than the energy provided by the food itself, you're not going to get the equivalent of a workout in by chomping on some celery sticks.

28

All it takes to lose weight is willpower.

Weight loss isn't as simple as willpower. If it were, then virtually everyone would be at their goal weight by now. Though part of losing weight is being able to control your impulses, genetics also play a role. "There are other more ignored parts that have to do with hormone and neurotransmitter imbalance," notes nutrition coach Teralyn Sell, PhD.

29

The scale is your only measurement of success.

During a weight loss journey, far too many people rely on the scale and the scale only to measure their success. In reality, your weight is constantly fluctuating, and so the number you see at any given point may not necessarily reflect your progress.

Instead of using the scale, Sell suggests that you "opt for a health measurement or [use] a non-scale victory to celebrate." By only paying minimal attention to the number on the scale, you can keep your mental health in check and avoid becoming "obsessed with every ounce, which can lead to more deprivation."

30

A raw food diet is a good way to lose weight.

Sure, a raw food diet is an effective way of losing weight—it's just not sustainable. In a 1999 study published in the Annals of Nutrition and Metabolism, researchers found that a strictly raw diet led to such a high degree of weight loss that it could not "be recommended on a long-term basis."

31

Going gluten-free increases weight loss.

A common misconception is that going gluten-free is a dieting decision. In reality, many people who nix gluten do so to avoid an inflammatory reaction in their immune systems. Unfortunately, eating gluten-free products with a weight loss goal in mind is bound to backfire.

"In many cases, the starchy wheat [in gluten-free products] is simply replaced by refined starches from rice, corn, or potato, which may not save you any calories," explains registered dietitian Susan Bowerman, senior director of worldwide nutrition education and training at Herbalife Nutrition. "Some gluten-free products also have a lot of added fat and sugar—often used to improve flavor or texture—so the calories can be very high."

32

Eating salad will help you slim down.

If all salads were created equal, this weight loss advice might hold true. But that's hardly the case. "One of the biggest problems with restaurant salads is that they're often overloaded with fat—and it isn't just from the dressing," explains Bowerman. "Other fatty add-ins like cheese, high-fat meats, fried tortilla strips or noodles, sour cream, and oily croutons can cause the calorie count to skyrocket."

33

If it's sold at the health food store, it's definitely good for you.

Branding can be deceiving. Just because something is sold at a health food store doesn't mean it's healthy. "There are plenty of high-sugar, high-fat items lurking on the shelves [at the health food store]," says Bowerman. "Are organic potato chips or sodas made with 'all-natural' sweeteners really any better for you than the regular stuff? Don't let the health halo fool you. Sticking with minimally processed foods is the best way to go—no matter where you shop."

34

Drinking too much water will make you bloated.

Most of us carry around some water weight—it's simply natural and shouldn't be considered "bloat." Besides, a 2015 study published in the journal Obesity found that drinking some extra water before meals actually increases weight loss. So drink up!

35

Drinking vinegar will increase your weight loss.

In additional to being foul-tasting, apple cider vinegar is an ineffective way to lose weight.

"When people overdo it, they get an upset stomach," notes registered dietitian Lisa Hugh.

36

Nuts are too high-calorie for most weight loss plans.

While nuts do tend to be calorie-rich, that doesn't mean they can't be effective parts of an overall weight loss plan. In fact, in a 2018 study published in the European Journal of Nutrition, researchers followed participants for five years and found that those who consumed the most nuts had less weight gain and a lower risk of being overweight than their peers who abstained. Nuts are a great source of healthy fat, so don't afraid to eat them in moderation.

37

Burning 3,500 calories equals a pound of weight lost.

The idea that burning or cutting 3,500 calories will necessarily result in a pound of weight loss is an outdated assumption that oversimplifies the complex processes involved in shedding pounds. The actual amount of weight loss achieved through a 3,500-calorie deficit is "substantially smaller" than predicted, according to a 2013 study in the New England Journal of Medicine.

38

Smoking is a good way to suppress your appetite.

This should go without saying, but cigarettes are not a diet tool. "Nicotine is an appetite suppressant, but risking your health for weight loss is not a good idea," says certified nutritionist Anju Mobin, managing editor of Best of Nutrition. "Smoking affects all organs of your body."

39

Skipping breakfast will boost your weight loss.

While skipping breakfast may indeed momentarily lower your calorie intake, it isn't a particularly effective long-term solution. In fact, one 2018 study presented at The Endocrine Society Annual Meeting found that eating a "high-energy breakfast"—meaning one that is large and calorie-rich—is a great way to spur weight loss. As bariatric surgeon Michael Russo, MD, explains, making breakfast your biggest meal "allows you to feel more energized throughout the day and allows your body the time to effectively utilize the calories instead of storing them while you sleep."

40

Multivitamins can make up for nutritional deficiencies when dieting.

Many multivitamins promise a quick fix for your long-term nutritional needs. However, a 2011 study published in the Journal of Agricultural and Food Chemistry reported that certain nutrients—once separated from the foods in which they are found—are less effective at providing the benefits they promise. In short, if you're in need of a vitamin or nutrient, go straight to the source.

41

Binge-eating is OK as long as you work out later.

"In reality, you can't make up for what happens in the kitchen at the gym," says Seti. "Nutritious foods can certainly fuel a good workout, but if you are looking to make up for what you've eaten, you would be in the gym hours upon hours each day to even come close to burning those calories."

42

You can only eat "bad foods" on cheat days.

Instead of having designated cheat days, you should allow yourself to indulge in your favorite foods whenever you please—just in moderation. "Telling yourself you can only eat the foods you want on a 'cheat' day makes it seem like you are doing something naughty or bad," explains registered dietitian Brittany Modell. "A sustainable diet is one that includes foods from all food groups seven days a week."

43

Using laxatives can help you shed pounds quickly.

Laxatives are not a weight loss tool, and they should only be used when medically necessary. According to the Nazarians, "using laxatives to lose weight is a terrible idea and can lead to a variety of medical issues such as dehydration, imbalances in electrolytes, and dependence."

44

Tummy-flattening teas are a great way to lose weight fast.

Don't believe everything you read on Kim Kardashian's Instagram. "There are lots of teas/drinks out there that market themselves as belly flatteners. A lot of them will make claims about working in 14 days or less, which is unrealistic and sets someone up for failure," notes registered dietitian nutritionist Jessi Holden, team lead for the Mary Free Bed Weight Management Program.

45

Every diet plan works the same for everybody.

"'One size fits all' diets are a bad idea," notes family nurse practitioner Tiffany Allen of Triad Lifestyle Medicine. "These plans don't take into account food sensitivities, budgets, preferences, and personality strengths and weaknesses." Everybody is different, and so what works for someone else might not necessarily work for you. It doesn't mean you're a failure—it just means you haven't found the right diet plan for you yet.

16/8 Intermittent Fasting: A Beginner's Guide

Fasting has been practiced for thousands of years and is a staple across many different religions and cultures around the globe.

Today, new varieties of fasting put a new twist on the ancient practice.

16/8 intermittent fasting is one of the most popular styles of fasting. Proponents claim that it's an easy, convenient and sustainable way to lose weight and improve overall health.

This article reviews 16/8 intermittent fasting, how it works and whether it's right for you.

What Is 16/8 Intermittent Fasting?

16/8 intermittent fasting involves limiting consumption of foods and calorie-containing beverages to a set window of eight hours per day and abstaining from food for the remaining 16 hours.

This cycle can be repeated as frequently as you like — from just once or twice per week to every day, depending on your personal preference.

16/8 intermittent fasting has skyrocketed in popularity in recent years, especially among those looking to lose weight and burn fat.

While other diets often set strict rules and regulations, 16/8 intermittent fasting is easy to follow and can provide real results with minimal effort.

It's generally considered less restrictive and more flexible than many other diet plans and can easily fit into just about any lifestyle.

In addition to enhancing weight loss, 16/8 intermittent fasting is also believed to improve blood sugar control, boost brain function and enhance longevity.

SUMMARY

16/8 intermittent fasting involves eating only during an eight-hour window during the day and fasting for the remaining 16 hours. It may support weight loss, improve blood sugar, boost brain function and increase longevity.

How to Get Started

16/8 intermittent fasting is simple, safe and sustainable.

To get started, begin by picking an eight-hour window and limit your food intake to that time span.

Many people prefer to eat between noon and 8 p.m., as this means you'll only need to fast overnight and skip breakfast but can still eat a balanced lunch and dinner, along with a few snacks throughout the day.

Others opt to eat between 9 a.m. and 5 p.m., which allows plenty of time for a healthy breakfast around 9 a.m., a normal lunch around noon and a light early dinner or snack around 4 p.m. before starting your fast.

However, you can experiment and pick the time frame that best fits your schedule.

Additionally, to maximize the potential health benefits of your diet, it's important to stick to nutritious whole foods and beverages during your eating periods.

Filling up on nutrient-rich foods can help round out your diet and allow you to reap the rewards that this regimen has to offer.

Try balancing each meal with a good variety of healthy whole foods, such as:

Fruits: Apples, bananas, berries, oranges, peaches, pears, etc.

Veggies: Broccoli, cauliflower, cucumbers, leafy greens, tomatoes, etc.

Whole grains: Quinoa, rice, oats, barley, buckwheat, etc.

Healthy fats: Olive oil, avocados and coconut oil

Sources of protein: Meat, poultry, fish, legumes, eggs, nuts, seeds, etc.

Drinking calorie-free beverages like water and unsweetened tea and coffee, even while fasting, can also help control your appetite while keeping you hydrated.

On the other hand, binging or overdoing it on junk food can negate the positive effects associated with 16/8 intermittent fasting and may end up doing more harm than good to your health.

Benefits of 16/8 Intermittent Fasting

16/8 intermittent fasting is a popular diet because it's easy to follow, flexible and sustainable in the long term.

It's also convenient, as it can cut down on the amount of time and money you need to spend on cooking and preparing food each week.

In terms of health, 16/8 intermittent fasting has been associated with a long list of benefits, including:

Increased weight loss: Not only does restricting your intake to a few hours per day help cut calories over the course of the day, but studies also show that fasting could boost metabolism and increase weight loss (1Trusted Source, 2Trusted Source).

Improved blood sugar control: Intermittent fasting has been found to reduce fasting insulin levels by up to 31% and lower blood sugar by 3–6%, potentially decreasing your risk of diabetes (2Trusted Source).

Enhanced longevity: Though evidence in humans is limited, some animal studies have found that intermittent fasting may extend longevity.

Drawbacks of 16/8 Intermittent Fasting

16/8 intermittent fasting may be associated with many health benefits, but it does come with some drawbacks and may not be right for everyone.

Restricting your intake to just eight hours per day can cause some people to eat more than usual during eating periods in an attempt to make up for hours spent fasting.

This may lead to weight gain, digestive problems and the development of unhealthy eating habits.

16/8 intermittent fasting may also cause short-term negative side effects when you're first getting started, such as hunger, weakness and fatigue — though these often subside once you get into a routine.

Additionally, some research suggests that intermittent fasting may affect men and women differently, with animal studies reporting that it could interfere with fertility and reproduction in females.

However, more human studies are needed to evaluate the effects that intermittent fasting may have on reproductive health.

In any case, be sure to start gradually and consider stopping or consulting your doctor if you have any concerns or experience negative symptoms.

SUMMARY

Restricting daily food intake may cause weakness, hunger, increased food consumption and weight gain. Animal studies show that intermittent fasting may impact men and women differently and may even interfere with fertility.

Is 16/8 Intermittent Fasting Right for You?

16/8 intermittent fasting can be a sustainable, safe and easy way to improve your health when paired with a nutritious diet and a healthy lifestyle.

However, it shouldn't be viewed as a substitute for a balanced, well-rounded diet rich in whole foods. Not to mention, you can still be healthy even if intermittent fasting doesn't work for you.

Though 16/8 intermittent fasting is generally considered safe for most healthy adults, you should talk to your doctor before giving it a try, especially if you have any underlying health conditions.

This is key if you're taking any medications or have diabetes, low blood pressure or a history of disordered eating.

Intermittent fasting is also not recommended for women who are trying to conceive or those who are pregnant or breastfeeding.

If you have any concerns or experience any adverse side effects while fasting, be sure to consult your doctor.

The Bottom Line

16/8 intermittent fasting involves eating only during an 8-hour window and fasting for the remaining 16 hours.

It may support weight loss and improve blood sugar, brain function and longevity.

Eat a healthy diet during your eating period and drink calorie-free beverages like water or unsweetened teas and coffee.

It's best to talk to your doctor before trying intermittent fasting, especially if you have any underlying health conditions.

People want to lose weight for a whole slew of different reasons. Some want to feel better about the way they look and give their self-esteem a boost, while others aim to stop using food as a coping mechanism for emotional struggles. No matter what reasons you have for...

YOU CAN DO IT TOO

CPSIA information can be obtained
at www.ICGtesting.com
Printed in the USA
BVHW091532150621
609534BV00002B/689